Dr. Jean Chapman

Effectively Maintaining Diabetes in Adults:

A Comprehensive Guide

Dr. Jean Chapman

Copyright @ 2022 Dr. Jean Chapman

Dr. Jean Chapman

Table of Contents

Introduction

Diabetes is a chronic condition that affects millions of adults worldwide. It requires careful management and maintenance to prevent complications and ensure a good quality of life. Regular monitoring of blood glucose levels, physical activity, proper diet, and timely medication are essential components of diabetes management. It is also important to be aware of the signs and symptoms of diabetes complications and to seek early medical attention if they develop. However, some people argue that diabetes is not a chronic condition. They argue that with proper diet and lifestyle changes, diabetes can be reversed. While this may be true for some people, it is not true for everyone. Diabetes is a chronic condition that requires lifelong management. In this comprehensive guide, we will explore various strategies and techniques for effectively maintaining diabetes in adults. By following these recommendations, individuals with diabetes can take charge of their health and minimize the impact of this condition on their daily lives. With the right lifestyle and medication, individuals with diabetes can manage their symptoms and lead a healthy and happy life. It is important to remember that diabetes is a serious condition, and it is essential to follow the recommendations of your healthcare provider to ensure proper management.

PART 1

Adopting a Healthy Lifestyle

The foundation of effective diabetes management lies in adopting a healthy lifestyle. Taking care of your body is similar to building a house; the foundations must be strong and secure to provide a safe and healthy environment. Adopting a healthy lifestyle is the basis of successful diabetes management. In another analogy, taking care of your body is like putting the pieces of a puzzle together. Each piece is an aspect of a healthy lifestyle that contributes to the overall picture. When all the pieces come together, it forms a strong and secure foundation that will support long-term health. This includes making informed dietary choices, engaging in regular physical activity, managing stress levels, and getting adequate sleep. A healthy lifestyle is a combination of all these pieces. Eating the right foods, exercising regularly, managing stress, and getting enough sleep are all essential components of a healthy lifestyle. When these pieces are combined, they create a strong foundation for long-term health. The components are therefore examined below;

a) Nutrition: A balanced diet is crucial for managing diabetes. Focus on consuming whole, unprocessed foods, including fruits, vegetables, lean proteins, and whole grains. Limit the intake of sugary beverages, refined carbohydrates, and saturated fats. Increase your intake of healthy fats, such as olive oil, nuts, and avocados. Drink plenty of water and get regular exercise. This lifestyle will help you maintain your blood sugar levels and reduce your risk of complications from diabetes. Consult a registered dietitian to create a personalized meal plan that meets your specific nutritional needs. This is similar to building a house; you need the right foundation, material, and tools to make sure it stands strong and lasts. Just like you need to properly construct a house, you need to carefully construct your diet to give your body the proper nourishment it needs to stay healthy and balanced.

b) **Physical Activity:** Regular exercise helps regulate blood sugar levels, improve insulin sensitivity, and maintain a healthy weight. Aim for at least 150 minutes of moderate-intensity aerobic activity per week and strength training exercises twice a week. Make sure to talk to your doctor before beginning any exercise program.

Start slowly and increase your intensity and duration gradually. Remember to rest between workouts to allow your body to fully recover. For instance, if you are new to exercise, start with 10-15 minutes of walking daily and gradually add more time and intensity to your routine. Make sure to listen to your body and adjust your routine accordingly. Change your exercise routine periodically to keep your body challenged and motivated. Don't forget to stay hydrated and eat a balanced diet to fuel your body.

c) Stress Management: Stress management is the ability to identify and cope with stressors in your life. There are many different stress management techniques, including exercise, relaxation, and time management. Stress management is like riding a bicycle: you have to learn to balance and steer, but the more you practice, the easier it becomes. By putting the tools into practice, you can gain the confidence to manage stress more effectively over time. For instance, a popular stress management technique is to practice mindfulness, which is focusing on the present moment and being aware of your thoughts, feelings, and environment. Chronic stress can negatively impact blood sugar control. Practice relaxation techniques such as deep breathing, meditation, or yoga to manage stress effectively. Of course, if none of this stress relieving techniques work, you can always just put on your favorite song and dance it out - it's the perfect way to let go of all your stress and worries!

d) Sleep: Sufficient sleep is essential for overall health and diabetes management. Aim for 7-9 hours of quality sleep each night. Establish a regular sleep routine and create a comfortable sleeping environment. Avoid caffeine and other stimulants close to bedtime. Exercise regularly but not too close to bedtime. Turn off electronic devices and dim the lights in the bedroom to help the body relax and prepare for sleep. Avoid large meals and alcohol close to bedtime. Practice relaxation techniques such as deep breathing, stretching, and mindfulness to help reduce stress and prepare for sleep. Create a bedtime routine and stick to it. On a lighter mode, set your alarm clock and put your bed back in its original place each morning! Ensure you get plenty of natural light during the day and avoid naps in the afternoon or evening. Also, make sure to get regular amounts of physical activity.

PART 2

Monitoring Blood Sugar Levels

Regular monitoring of blood sugar levels is essential for effective diabetes management. This provides valuable information to adjust treatment plans and prevent complications. Additionally, it can help people with diabetes to understand how their diet and lifestyle choices affect their condition. Monitoring blood sugar levels regularly can also help to identify any early warning signs of changes in health. The American Diabetes Association's goals for blood sugar control in people with diabetes are 70 to 130 mg/dL before meals and less than 180 mg/dL after meals. Regular monitoring and following the ADA's guidelines can help people with diabetes to better manage their condition and maintain their health. The following are key elements of blood sugar monitoring:

a) **Self-Monitoring:** Use a blood glucose meter to measure blood sugar levels at home. It can take up to 3 months to see significant changes in your A1C levels. Record the results in a logbook. If readings are too high or too low, contact your healthcare team. They can provide advice and adjust your treatment plan if necessary. For instance, if your blood sugar levels are too high, your healthcare team may recommend increasing your insulin dosage or changing your meal plan. Follow the recommended frequency and timing as advised by your healthcare provider. Check your feet regularly for blisters, sores, redness, or swelling. Test your urine for ketones when your blood sugar is high. Monitor your blood pressure and cholesterol levels regularly. Keep a record of these readings to identify patterns and discuss them during medical appointments. Oh and don't forget to take a break and watch your favorite sitcom every once in awhile - it's always a good idea to laugh and de-stress!

b) **Continuous Glucose Monitoring (CGM):** CGM devices provide real-time glucose readings throughout the day. This allows users to get an accurate picture of their glucose levels and to make adjustments to their diet and lifestyle accordingly. CGM technology is especially helpful for people with diabetes or other conditions that require frequent monitoring of blood sugar levels. It can be a valuable tool for managing diabetes and improving quality of life. CGM devices also alert users when their glucose levels reach certain thresholds, allowing them to take appropriate action to stabilize their blood sugar levels. This can help prevent serious health complications and improve overall health outcomes. They offer a more comprehensive understanding of blood sugar fluctuations and trends. Using a CGM device to monitor and manage diabetes is similar to a pilot having access to instrumentation and dashboard warnings that help them avoid turbulence and dangerous weather. The data helps the pilot stay on course and reach their destination safely. Similarly, CGM devices can help people with diabetes understand their blood sugar levels and take steps to adjust their diet and lifestyle accordingly. With this data, they can stay healthy and avoid dangerous blood sugar levels. However, consult with your healthcare provider to determine if a CGM device is suitable for you.

c) **Glycated Hemoglobin (HbA1c):** HbA1c test measures average blood sugar levels over the past 2-3 months. It is used to diagnose diabetes and to monitor the effectiveness of diabetes treatment.

HbA1c results are expressed as a percentage. Results of 6.5% or higher indicate diabetes. It provides a broader perspective on long-term glucose control. Aim for a target HbA1c level as recommended by your healthcare provider. Regular HbA1c tests can help to detect diabetes when it is still in the early stages. It can also help to adjust treatments when needed, to ensure that the diabetes is under control. HbA1c testing should be done regularly as recommended by your healthcare provider. It's like taking a car for regular maintenance checks - if you don't have regular tests, you won't know when something is wrong until it's too late. Regular tests are necessary to keep the car running smoothly and prevent bigger problems from arising down the road. Just like when you ignore the "check engine" light for too long and suddenly you're stranded on the side of the road. Don't let that be you and your diabetes! Get your HbA1c test done regularly so you don't end up in a sticky situation.

PART 3

Medication management

In addition to lifestyle modifications, medication plays a vital role in managing diabetes. Medications can help lower blood sugar levels, reduce the risk of complications, and improve overall health and quality of life. It is imperative to take medications as prescribed and to work closely with a healthcare provider to monitor and adjust medications as needed. Taking diabetes medications is similar to taking a vitamin or other supplement—it's an added layer of protection that can help keep your body healthier and functioning as it should. It's an important part of your health care plan that is necessary for successful management of diabetes. Here are some common medications used to treat diabetes:

a) **Insulin:** Insulin therapy is typically prescribed for individuals with type 1 diabetes and some with type 2 diabetes. Insulin helps regulate the blood sugar levels of individuals with diabetes. It is taken either through injections or an insulin pump. Monitoring and maintaining healthy blood sugar levels is an important part of managing diabetes. Taking insulin is similar to a thermostat in a home, it helps to regulate the temperature of the environment to maintain a balance. In the same way, insulin helps to regulate and balance blood sugar levels to prevent drastic swings that can have negative health consequences. It helps regulate blood sugar levels by replacing or supplementing the body's insulin production. Currently, it is estimated that 37.3 million Americans have diabetes, which equals about 1 in 10 people. With this high number of diabetic patients, Insulin tends to be a life-saving medication for people with diabetes, and it is important to take insulin as prescribed by a healthcare provider. Without insulin, people with diabetes would be at risk for developing serious health complications such as heart disease, stroke, and kidney failure.

b) **Oral Medications:** Several classes of oral medications are available for type 2 diabetes. These include metformin, sulfonylureas, DPP-4 inhibitors, SGLT2 inhibitors, and others. They work by improving insulin sensitivity, reducing glucose production, or enhancing insulin release. They can also be used in combination with other medications, including insulin, to help achieve better glycemic control. However, they can also cause side effects such as weight gain, nausea, and low blood sugar. Patients should discuss the benefits and risks with their doctor before taking these medications. These medications are usually prescribed when lifestyle changes such as diet and exercise are not enough to control blood sugar levels. They help to regulate blood sugar levels by increasing the body's sensitivity to insulin, reducing the amount of glucose produced by the liver, or increasing the amount of insulin released by the pancreas.

c) **Other Injectable Medications:** GLP-1 receptor agonists, such as exenatide and liraglutide, are injectable medications that help control blood sugar levels by stimulating insulin release and suppressing glucagon secretion. GLP-1 receptor agonists also slow the rate of digestion and reduce appetite, which can lead to weight loss. These medications are usually administered once or twice a day and are generally well tolerated. For instance, exenatide is typically administered subcutaneously twice daily, while liraglutide is usually administered as a once-daily injection. GLP-1 receptor agonists have been shown to be effective in lowering blood sugar levels and improving glycemic control in people with type 2 diabetes. They can also be used to treat obesity in people who have not achieved adequate weight loss through lifestyle modifications.

END NOTE

Summarily, effective diabetes management requires a holistic approach that combines healthy lifestyle practices, regular blood sugar monitoring, and appropriate medication management. It is important to work with a healthcare provider to develop a diabetes management plan. With the right plan, people with diabetes can lead healthy, active lives. It is also important to stay informed about advances in diabetes treatments. By adopting these strategies, individuals with diabetes can lead fulfilling lives while minimizing the risk of complications. Remember to work closely with your healthcare provider to develop a personalized diabetes management plan that suits your specific needs. Together, you can navigate the challenges of diabetes and maintain optimal health and well-being.

www.ingramcontent.com/pod-product-compliance
Lightning Source LLC
Chambersburg PA
CBHW060906260726
48661CB00008B/3481